Harness Nature's Cure:
Health Benefits of Ginger

Ginger Remedy:
A Comprehensive Guide to Unlocking the Healing Power Within

JAMES BRANDY

TABLE OF CONTENTS

INTRODUCTION

Unlocking the Healing Power of Ginger

In a world where the pursuit of wellness is both timeless and ever-evolving, nature's remedies continue to hold a profound allure. Among these, ginger stands as a beacon of healing, revered across centuries and continents for its remarkable therapeutic properties. In this exploration of the healing power of ginger, we embark on a journey that transcends the confines of conventional medicine to unveil the profound potential of this humble rhizome.

Ginger, with its fiery taste and invigorating aroma, has long captivated the senses and captured the imagination of healers and herbalists alike. From ancient civilizations to modern laboratories, the story of ginger unfolds as a testament to the enduring symbiosis between humanity and nature. It is a story woven with threads of tradition, innovation, and a deep reverence for the intrinsic wisdom of the natural world.

In the pages that follow, we delve into the multifaceted facets of ginger's healing prowess, exploring its role in nurturing physical, mental, and emotional well-being. From its soothing effects on digestive discomfort to its potential to alleviate pain and inflammation, ginger emerges as a versatile ally in the quest for holistic health. But beyond its tangible benefits lies a deeper narrative—a narrative of cultural richness, culinary creativity, and a timeless connection to the rhythms of the earth.

As we navigate the realms of science, tradition, and personal experience, we invite you to embark on this odyssey of discovery. Whether you are a seasoned herbalist or a curious seeker, "The Healing Power of Ginger" offers insights, inspiration, and practical guidance to empower your wellness journey. It is a celebration of the extraordinary potential nestled within a seemingly ordinary root—a reminder that the most profound remedies are often found in the simplest of gifts from nature.

So, join us as we unlock the healing power of ginger, one revelation at a time. Let this journey be a testament to the enduring bond between humanity and the natural world—and may it inspire you to cultivate a deeper connection with the healing wonders that surround us.

Section 1: Anatomy of the Ginger Plant

As we embark on this journey of discovery, it's imperative to acquaint ourselves with the very essence of our subject – the ginger plant. In this section, we delve into the intricate anatomy that forms the foundation of ginger's botanical brilliance.

Ginger, scientifically known as Zingiber officinale, is not just a root but a complex network of rhizomes, stems, and leaves. We will unravel the layers of this botanical marvel, exploring how each component contributes to the plant's vitality and the unique compounds that make it a powerhouse of health.

From the subterranean rhizomes, the source of ginger's distinctive flavor and medicinal properties, to the towering stems that bear the lush foliage, understanding the anatomy of the ginger plant provides a holistic perspective. Appreciate the synergy between roots and shoots, and grasp how this balance is harnessed for both culinary and therapeutic purposes.

Section 2: Types and Varieties

Ginger is a diverse botanical family with various types and varieties that have adapted to different climates and regions. In this section, we embark on a global tour, exploring the nuances that distinguish one ginger variety from another.

From the piquant and citrusy Jamaican ginger to the robust and earthy Indian varieties, each type carries its unique flavor profile and potential health benefits. Delve into the cultivation practices that influence the characteristics of different gingers and learn how to discern between them.

Understanding the types and varieties of ginger not only enhances your culinary experiences but also allows you to make informed choices when seeking specific health benefits. Join us on this exploration of diversity within the ginger family, as we unravel the tapestry of flavors and therapeutic potentials that make each variety a botanical masterpiece.

CHAPTER TWO

Nutritional Breakdown

Section 1: Essential Nutrients in Ginger

As we peel back the layers of ginger's nutritional profile, we uncover a treasure trove of essential nutrients that contribute to its remarkable healing properties. In this section, we dissect the components that make ginger not just a culinary delight but also a powerhouse of health.

Explore the wealth of vitamins and minerals nestled within the fibrous structure of ginger. From the immune-boosting vitamin C to the bone-strengthening magnesium, each nutrient plays a crucial role in supporting overall well-being. Unravel the intricate dance of antioxidants that help combat oxidative stress, protecting your cells from damage and promoting longevity.

Beyond the commonly recognized nutrients, ginger also houses bioactive compounds like gingerol, responsible for its distinctive flavor and potent medicinal effects. Gain insights into how these compounds interact with your body, influencing everything from inflammation to digestion.

Section 2: Dietary Benefits

The benefits of incorporating ginger into your diet extend far beyond its flavorful punch. In this section, we explore how integrating this rhizome into your meals can be a proactive step toward enhancing your health.

Dive into the digestive benefits as ginger aids in alleviating nausea, soothing indigestion, and promoting a healthy gut microbiome. Uncover its anti-inflammatory properties, which can play a pivotal role in managing chronic conditions and supporting joint health.

But the advantages of ginger are not limited to the physical; we also delve into its potential impact on mental well-being. From cognitive support to stress reduction, discover how the compounds within ginger contribute to a holistic sense of vitality.

Join us as we navigate the nutritional labyrinth of ginger, demystifying the elements that make it not just a spice but a nutritional powerhouse. Through a deeper understanding of essential nutrients and dietary benefits, you'll be equipped to harness ginger's full potential for your health and wellness journey.

CHAPTER THREEE

The Science Behind the Magic

Section 1: Phytochemicals and Their Impact

Ginger boasts a rich array of phytochemicals, including gingerol, shogaol, and parasols, each contributing uniquely to its medicinal effects. We decipher how these compounds interact with cellular processes, acting as antioxidants and anti-inflammatory agents. Through this exploration, gain insights into the intricate dance of molecules that make ginger a natural remedy for various ailments.

Understanding the phytochemical fingerprint of ginger not only enhances your appreciation for its complexity but also empowers you to harness its benefits consciously. From its aromatic essence to its therapeutic depth, each phytochemical plays a role in unlocking the magic within.

Section 2: Ginger's Role in Inflammation and Immunity

The synergy of ginger's bioactive compounds manifests prominently in its role in managing inflammation and bolstering the immune system. In this section, we dissect the mechanisms through which ginger becomes a guardian of your body's defense and healing mechanisms.

Explore how ginger's anti-inflammatory properties can mitigate chronic inflammation, a common underlying factor in various diseases. From joint pain to cardiovascular health, we uncover the breadth of conditions where ginger's influence is felt.

Delve into the immune-modulating effects of ginger, understanding how it can fortify your body's natural defenses. From its antimicrobial properties to its role in maintaining a balanced immune response, ginger emerges as a versatile ally in the pursuit of overall well-being.

Join us as we navigate the intricate pathways of ginger's scientific enchantment, unveiling the mechanisms that make it not just a spice but a profound contributor to your health journey. Through this exploration, you'll gain a deeper appreciation for the symbiotic relationship between ginger and the human body.

CHAPTER FOUR

Culinary Uses

Section 1: Incorporating Ginger into Your Diet

Embark on a culinary adventure as we explore the art of seamlessly integrating ginger into your daily meals. In this section, we unravel the secrets of making ginger a versatile and delectable addition to your diet.

Discover the myriad ways to incorporate fresh and ground ginger into various dishes, from breakfast to dinner. Whether it's infusing beverages with a zingy flavor or adding a hint of warmth to desserts, the possibilities are as diverse as the culinary traditions that embrace this spice.

Explore cooking techniques that maximize ginger's flavor and nutritional benefits. From stir-frying to slow simmering, learn how to enhance the taste profile of your dishes while preserving the integrity of this remarkable rhizome.

Section 2: Delicious Recipes for Health

Turn your kitchen into a haven of health with a collection of mouthwatering recipes designed to make ginger the star of your meals. From appetizers to main courses and even desserts, each recipe is crafted not only for flavor but also for its potential health benefits.

Ginger-Infused Green Tea: Elevate your tea time with the refreshing combination of green tea and a hint of ginger, packed with antioxidants and digestive benefits.

Spiced Carrot and Ginger Soup: Immerse yourself in the comfort of a warming bowl of soup, where the natural sweetness of carrots meets the kick of ginger for a nutrient-rich delight.

Grilled Salmon with Ginger Glaze: Transform a simple salmon dish into a culinary masterpiece by infusing it with a ginger glaze that not only enhances the flavor but also adds anti-inflammatory properties.

Ginger Turmeric Smoothie: Kickstart your day with a vibrant and immune-boosting smoothie, blending the goodness of ginger with turmeric and other wholesome ingredients.

Mango Ginger Sorbet: Indulge your sweet tooth guilt-free with a refreshing sorbet that combines the tropical sweetness of mango with the invigorating essence of ginger.

Through these recipes, you'll not only savor the culinary delights but also experience the healthful benefits that come with embracing ginger as a staple in your kitchen. Join us on this culinary exploration, where the marriage of flavor and well-being takes center stage.

Section 1: Homemade Ginger Infusions

Unlock the therapeutic potential of ginger within the confines of your kitchen with this exploration into homemade infusions. In this section, we delve into the art of crafting ginger-infused elixirs that not only tantalize your taste buds but also nurture your well-being.

Ginger Tea Elixir: Learn the art of brewing the perfect cup of ginger tea, a comforting and aromatic beverage known for its digestive benefits and immune-boosting properties.

Honey-Ginger Syrup: Elevate your sweeteners by creating a versatile honey-ginger syrup. Drizzle it over desserts, add it to beverages, or simply enjoy a spoonful for a delightful fusion of flavors with potential health perks.

Ginger Lemonade with a Twist: Refresh your senses with a zesty ginger-infused lemonade. Perfect for hot days, this beverage not only quenches your thirst but also provides a burst of antioxidants.

Explore the diverse world of ginger infusions, where each concoction is a unique blend of flavors and potential health benefits. From soothing stomach woes to boosting your immune system, these homemade infusions offer a holistic approach to well-being.

Section 2: External Applications for Wellness

Extend the healing touch of ginger beyond the internal realm and explore its efficacy in external applications. In this section, we uncover how ginger's properties can be harnessed topically for various wellness purposes.

Ginger Compress for Pain Relief: Craft a soothing ginger compress to alleviate muscle soreness and joint pain. The warming effect of ginger can provide comfort and relaxation when applied externally.

Ginger Hair Mask: Nourish your hair and scalp with a homemade ginger hair mask. Known for its potential to stimulate blood circulation, ginger may contribute to healthier hair growth.

Ginger-Infused Bath Soak: Transform your bath into a spa-like experience with a ginger-infused bath soak. Immerse yourself in the aromatic warmth that ginger brings, promoting relaxation and easing tension.

By exploring the external applications of ginger, you'll discover how this versatile rhizome can play a role in enhancing your overall well-being, both inside and out. Join us in this hands-on journey of DIY ginger remedies, where the power to heal is at your fingertips.

CHAPTER SIX

Ginger in Traditional Medicine

Section 1: Historical Uses Across Cultures

Embark on a journey through time and space as we uncover the rich tapestry of ginger's historical significance in traditional medicine across diverse cultures. In this section, we explore the roots of ginger's therapeutic reputation and its enduring presence in ancient healing practices.

Ancient China: The Herb of Harmony: Trace ginger's origins in traditional Chinese medicine, where it earned a reputation as a balancing herb, used to harmonize bodily functions and promote overall wellness.

Ayurveda in India: The Universal Medicine: Delve into the pages of Ayurveda, where ginger is hailed as an indispensable herb. From digestive aid to respiratory support, discover how Ayurvedic practitioners have valued ginger for its holistic healing properties.

Middle Eastern Traditions: A Culinary and Medicinal Delight: Uncover the multifaceted role of ginger in Middle Eastern traditions, where it transcended the kitchen to become a staple in herbal remedies for various ailments.

Section 2: Folk Remedies and Wisdom

Explore the wisdom passed down through generations as communities around the world incorporated ginger into their folk remedies. In this section, we delve into the diverse ways ginger has been utilized in homes and villages, guided by the collective knowledge of generations.

Ginger for Digestive Harmony: Unearth the folk remedies that have long used ginger as a digestive aid, addressing issues from indigestion to nausea, passed down through the oral traditions of communities worldwide.

Ginger for Cold and Flu: Discover the age-old wisdom of using ginger to combat respiratory ailments. From teas to poultices, explore how ginger has been a trusted ally in the fight against common colds and flu-like symptoms.

Ginger in Women's Health: Examine the traditional applications of ginger in addressing women's health concerns, from menstrual discomfort to pregnancy-related nausea, drawing upon the wisdom of generations of healers.

By understanding the historical roots and folk wisdom surrounding ginger in traditional medicine, we gain profound insights into the enduring reverence for this remarkable rhizome. Join us as we navigate the crossroads of time and tradition, exploring the universal recognition of ginger as a valuable asset in the pursuit of health and well-being.

Section 1: Alleviating Digestive Discomfort

Embark on a journey into the soothing realms of ginger as we explore its remarkable ability to alleviate digestive discomfort. In this section, we unravel the digestive mysteries that ginger addresses, offering relief and promoting overall gastrointestinal well-being.

Calming the Upset Stomach: Explore how ginger has been a time-tested remedy for soothing an upset stomach. Whether it's indigestion, bloating, or general discomfort, ginger's natural properties can provide gentle relief.

Nausea and Motion Sickness: Uncover the science behind ginger's anti-nausea properties, examining its effectiveness in addressing everything from morning sickness to motion-induced queasiness. Discover the various forms in which ginger can be consumed to ease nausea.

Ginger for Digestive Harmony: Delve into how ginger supports overall digestive harmony. From enhancing the production of digestive enzymes to promoting a healthy gut microbiome, explore the multifaceted role ginger plays in optimizing digestion.

Section 2: Gut-Healing Properties

Explore the deeper layers of ginger's impact on digestive health, delving into its potential as a gut-healing ally. In this section, we uncover the mechanisms through which ginger contributes to a resilient and thriving gastrointestinal system.

Anti-Inflammatory Action in the Gut: Examine how ginger's anti-inflammatory properties extend to the digestive tract, potentially mitigating inflammation associated with conditions such as irritable bowel syndrome (IBS) and inflammatory bowel diseases (IBD).

Balancing Gut Microbiota: Discover the prebiotic-like effects of ginger, which may foster the growth of beneficial gut bacteria. Explore the intricate interplay between ginger and the microbiome, and how this synergy contributes to digestive well-being.

Ginger and Intestinal Permeability: Delve into the potential role of ginger in supporting a healthy intestinal barrier. Explore how this aspect of ginger's properties may contribute to managing conditions associated with increased intestinal permeability, such as leaky gut syndrome.

Join us as we navigate the digestive landscape, uncovering how ginger emerges as a soothing balm for discomfort and a proactive agent in fostering gut health. Through this exploration, you'll gain insights into how ginger can become a valuable ally in your journey toward a balanced and resilient digestive system.

Section 1: Natural Pain Relief

Embark on a journey into the realm of natural pain relief as we explore how ginger, with its time-honored reputation, can be a valuable ally in managing various types of pain. In this section, we delve into how ginger serves as a gentle yet potent alternative to conventional pain management.

Headaches and Migraines: Explore the potential of ginger in alleviating tension headaches and migraines. Uncover how its anti-inflammatory and vasodilatory properties may contribute to relief from headaches.

Muscle and Joint Pain: Delve into the soothing effects of ginger on muscle and joint pain. Whether it's post-exercise soreness or chronic conditions like arthritis, discover how ginger's natural compounds may offer comfort and flexibility.

Menstrual Pain: Examine the role of ginger in addressing menstrual pain. From cramps to discomfort, explore how incorporating ginger into your routine may provide a natural and holistic approach to menstrual pain relief.

Section 2: Combating Inflammation

Uncover the intricate relationship between ginger and inflammation, a key factor in various types of pain. In this section, we explore how ginger's anti-inflammatory properties make it a powerful tool in combating pain associated with inflammation.

Understanding Inflammation: Gain insights into the basics of inflammation and how it contributes to pain. Explore the role of chronic inflammation in conditions like arthritis and how ginger's compounds may help modulate inflammatory responses.

Ginger's Anti-Inflammatory Mechanisms: Delve into the specific mechanisms through which ginger combats inflammation. From inhibiting inflammatory mediators to suppressing oxidative stress, explore how ginger's multifaceted approach may contribute to reducing pain.

Chronic Pain Conditions: Explore the potential applications of ginger in managing chronic pain conditions. Whether it's osteoarthritis, rheumatoid arthritis, or other inflammatory disorders, discover how ginger's natural properties offer hope for those seeking alternative pain management solutions.

Join us as we navigate the realm of pain management, uncovering the natural pathways through which ginger emerges as a beacon of relief. Through this exploration, you'll gain insights into how ginger can become a valuable companion in your journey toward a more comfortable and pain-free life.

Section 1: Cognitive Benefits

Embark on a journey into the realm of cognitive enhancement as we explore the potential of ginger to support mental well-being. In this section, we unravel the cognitive benefits that ginger offers, contributing to mental clarity and overall brain health.

Memory and Focus: Dive into how ginger may positively influence memory and concentration. Explore the potential neuroprotective effects of ginger's bioactive compounds and their impact on cognitive function.

Mood and Emotional Well-being: Uncover the connections between ginger and mood regulation. From its potential role in serotonin modulation to its overall impact on emotional well-being, explore how ginger may contribute to a positive mental state.

Neurological Health: Examine the potential neuroprotective properties of ginger. From its antioxidant effects to its role in reducing neuroinflammation, discover how ginger may play a part in safeguarding the health of your nervous system.

Section 2: Stress Reduction and Relaxation

Explore the soothing side of ginger as we delve into its role in stress reduction and relaxation. In this section, we uncover how ginger's calming properties may offer respite amid life's pressures.

Adaptogenic Qualities: Understand how ginger may act as an adaptogen, helping the body adapt to stress and maintain balance. Explore the potential of ginger in supporting the adrenal glands and mitigating the physiological effects of stress.

Relaxation and Sleep: Delve into the calming effects of ginger on the nervous system. Explore how ginger may contribute to relaxation, potentially aiding in better sleep quality and managing sleep-related issues.

Stress-Induced Ailments: Examine how ginger may alleviate ailments exacerbated by stress. From tension headaches to gastrointestinal issues, discover how ginger's dual action on cognitive and physiological aspects may offer a holistic approach to stress management.

Join us on this exploration of ginger's impact on mental well-being, where cognitive benefits and stress reduction converge to provide a comprehensive perspective on how ginger can become a supportive element in your journey toward a balanced and resilient mind.

Section 1: Maintaining Cardiovascular Wellness

Embark on a heart-healthy journey with ginger as we explore its potential to maintain cardiovascular wellness. In this section, we delve into how ginger contributes to a healthy heart, fostering overall cardiovascular well-being.

Cholesterol Regulation: Uncover the potential of ginger in positively influencing cholesterol levels. Explore how ginger's compounds may contribute to reducing LDL cholesterol and triglycerides, promoting a more heart-healthy lipid profile.

Antioxidant Protection: Delve into the antioxidant properties of ginger and their impact on cardiovascular health. Explore how ginger's ability to combat oxidative stress may play a role in preventing the oxidation of LDL cholesterol and reducing the risk of atherosclerosis.

Anti-Inflammatory Effects on the Heart: Understand the connection between inflammation and heart health. Explore how ginger's anti-inflammatory properties may contribute to reducing inflammation in the cardiovascular system, potentially lowering the risk of heart disease.

Section 2: Managing Blood Pressure

Explore the potential of ginger in managing blood pressure, a crucial aspect of cardiovascular health. In this section, we unravel how ginger may play a role in maintaining healthy blood pressure levels.

Vasodilation and Blood Flow: Delve into how ginger may influence blood vessel function. Explore the potential of ginger in promoting vasodilation, improving blood flow, and contributing to healthy blood pressure regulation.

Antihypertensive Properties: Uncover the potential antihypertensive effects of ginger. Explore how ginger's bioactive compounds may act as natural ACE inhibitors, potentially helping to lower blood pressure and manage hypertension.

Stress Reduction and Heart Health: Examine the relationship between stress, blood pressure, and heart health. Discover how ginger's adaptogenic qualities may contribute to stress reduction, potentially benefiting blood pressure management and overall cardiovascular wellness.

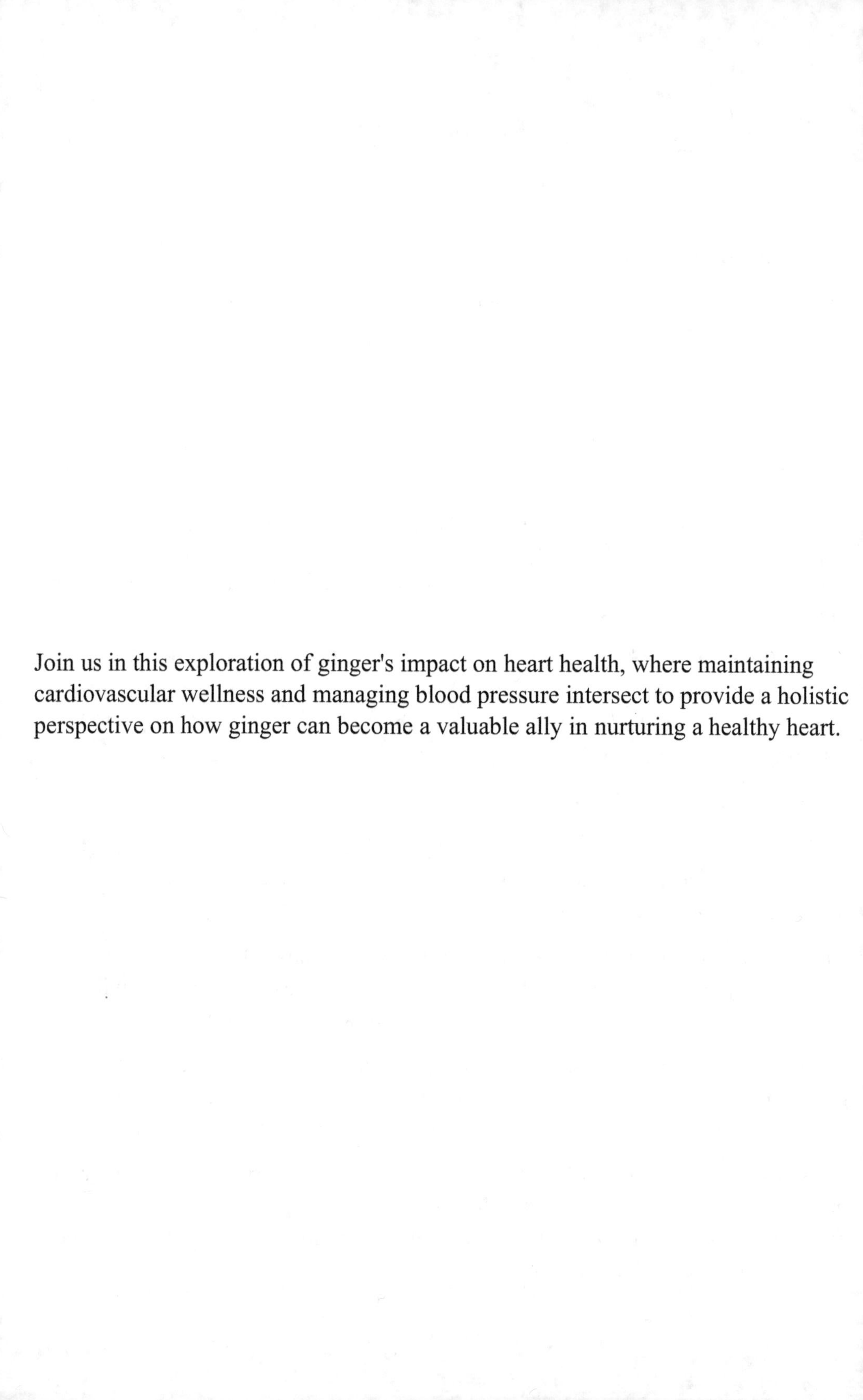

Join us in this exploration of ginger's impact on heart health, where maintaining cardiovascular wellness and managing blood pressure intersect to provide a holistic perspective on how ginger can become a valuable ally in nurturing a healthy heart.

Section 1: Ongoing Studies

Embark on a journey into the future as we explore the ongoing studies that continue to unravel the mysteries and potentials of ginger. In this section, we delve into the current research initiatives that are shaping the landscape of ginger's role in health and wellness.

Ginger and Neurological Health: Investigate the ongoing studies exploring the potential neuroprotective effects of ginger. From cognitive enhancement to neurological disorders, researchers are delving into how ginger may play a role in safeguarding the health of the brain.

Ginger and Cardiovascular Benefits: Explore the evolving research on ginger's impact on cardiovascular health. Ongoing studies are examining its potential in preventing heart disease, managing risk factors, and contributing to overall cardiovascular wellness.

Ginger's Role in Metabolic Health: Delve into the research focused on ginger's influence on metabolic health. From blood sugar regulation to potential implications for conditions like diabetes, ongoing studies aim to uncover the nuanced interactions between ginger and metabolic processes.

Section 2: Potential Discoveries

Anticipate the potential discoveries that may reshape our understanding of ginger and its applications in health and wellness. In this section, we explore the exciting possibilities that future research may unveil.

Ginger and Immune Modulation: Envision the potential for ginger to modulate immune responses. Emerging research may shed light on how ginger's compounds interact with the immune system, influencing both innate and adaptive immunity.

Ginger's Impact on Microbiome: Explore the potential discoveries related to ginger's influence on the gut microbiome. Ongoing research may reveal how ginger interacts with gut bacteria, contributing to a balanced and thriving microbial environment.

Precision Medicine and Ginger: Envision a future where ginger is personalized for individual health needs. Research may uncover genetic factors that influence how individuals respond to ginger, paving the way for precision medicine approaches.

As we peer into the future of ginger research, the possibilities are vast and promising. Join us in this exploration of ongoing studies and potential discoveries, where the evolving landscape of ginger's therapeutic potential continues to unfold.

CONCLUSION

In the culmination of our exploration into the versatile world of ginger, let's reflect on the key takeaways that empower your health journey.

Holistic Healing: Ginger transcends its culinary allure, emerging as a holistic healer. From digestive well-being to cognitive health, its multifaceted properties offer a comprehensive approach to wellness.

Ancient Wisdom, Modern Science: Bridging the wisdom of ancient traditions with contemporary research, ginger stands as a testament to the enduring synergy between time-honored practices and scientific advancements.

Culinary Creativity: The kitchen becomes your sanctuary as you learn to incorporate ginger into diverse culinary creations. From soothing teas to delectable dishes, the art of using ginger becomes an empowering aspect of your daily life.

Natural Remedies: Dive into the world of DIY ginger remedies, discovering how simple infusions and external applications can be powerful tools for self-care, offering relief and promoting overall well-being.

Cultural Richness: Explore ginger's cultural significance, traversing continents and traditions. From ancient Chinese herbalism to Middle Eastern culinary delights, ginger weaves a rich tapestry of cultural connections.

Versatile Ally: Ginger emerges as a versatile ally in managing pain, supporting mental well-being, and nurturing cardiovascular health. Its adaptogenic qualities and anti-inflammatory properties make it a valuable companion on your health journey.

Ongoing Exploration: As we glimpse into the future, ongoing studies and potential discoveries hint at a deeper understanding of ginger's therapeutic potential. The journey with ginger is dynamic, with continuous revelations shaping its role in the evolving landscape of health and wellness.

In empowering your health journey with ginger, may you savor not only its distinctive flavor but also the profound benefits it offers. Whether you seek comfort in a cup of ginger tea, explore its culinary versatility, or delve into the realms of natural remedies, let ginger be your companion on the path to holistic well-being. Cheers to a vibrant and healthful life, enriched by the magic of ginger.